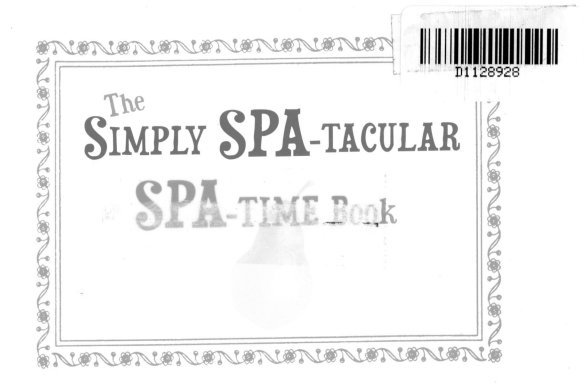

The SIMPLY SPA-TACULAR SPA-TIME Book

Pamper and soothe yourself and your friends with over **30 SPA**-time activities, recipes, and party ideas.

Erin Conley and Jennifer Worick

Photography by Julie Brown

Illustrations by Annie Galvin

7

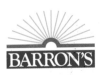

BARRON'S

THE SIMPLY SPA-TACULAR SPA-TIME BOOK

First edition for the United States and Canada published in 2004
by Barron's Educational Series, Inc.

Created and produced by Orange Avenue Publishing, San Francisco, CA.
© 2004 by Orange Avenue Publishing
Illustrations © 2004 by Annie Galvin
Photographs © 2004 by Julie Brown

All inquiries should be addressed to:
Barron's Educational Series, Inc.
250 Wireless Boulevard
Hauppauge, NY 11788
http://www.barronseduc.com

Library of Congress Catalog Card No. 2003108849

International Standard Book No. 0-7641-2574-5

Printed in China

9 8 7 6 5 4 3 2 1

The SIMPLY SPA-TACULAR SPA-TIME Book

Contents

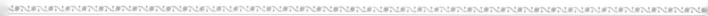

The SPA Story

In the Beginning...

Many, many years before the modern-day spa was born, stressed-out and health-savvy citizens in ancient Europe gathered at public baths, steam rooms, and saunas to relax and reconnect. They'd soothe their spirits and heal their bodies with warm baths, massage, and (most importantly) the company of good friends.

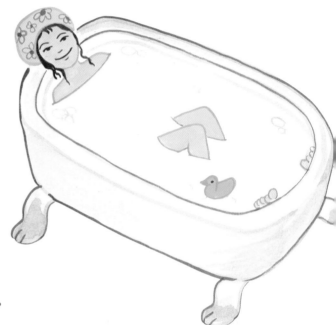

And then there was the SPA...

Although the focus is still on inner bliss, spas have evolved quite a bit. Some spa hot spots have even achieved celebrity status! People have flocked to Bath, England, for thousands of years to take a dip in its warm waters. The Dead Sea, one of the saltiest lakes in the world, is another popular spot with people who like to cover themselves in its famous mud. Whatever your pampering preference, there is at least one spa treatment that is sure to rejuvenate and relax your soul.

And now there is The SIMPLY SPA-TACULAR SPA-TIME BOOK!

This book celebrates 16 fun-filled spa varieties and includes easy-to-make recipes for spa drinks and snacks. Find your inner "om" with an outside yoga class, kick back and enjoy a yogurt *Spa*rfait, or create and bottle yummy lotions, (complete with your own logo and fancy labels). But most importantly, discover that being beautiful is about feeling good rather than just looking good. It's about treating yourself – and others – well.

So gather your girlfriends, a sense of adventure, and a creative spirit. You'll need them all to concoct each of the delicious treats we have in store for your mind, body, and belly. Now take a deep breath, let your hair down, and begin rubbing, massaging, polishing, painting, stretching, eating, drinking, and *spa*rtying for a total head-to-toe glow!

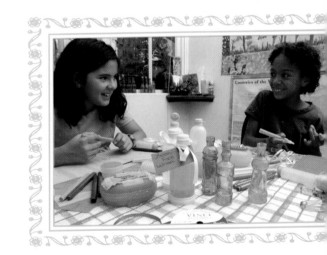

SPA BASICS

Get ready to relax! Whether you're the hostess with the mostess or a pampered guest, it's important to sound – as well as feel – calm, cool, and collected at a *spa*rty. Check out the glossary below to brush up on some of the posh lingo for those oh-so exclusive treatments. That way you'll know exactly what treats you're in for!

Aromatherapy: This popular technique uses essential oils to soothe your mind and your body. Some massages include aromatherapy, but you can also simply take a whiff of a particular scent to mellow, enliven, heal – or whatever your spirit needs!

Carrier Oil: Sounds contagious, but it's actually just a harmless, moisturizing oil (like olive or sweet almond oil). Add a few drops of one of these to your favorite essential oil to make the scent subtler.

Cleanse: This is another way of saying, "Wash your face, girl!" You may have heard your mom or big sister throw this term around.

Cuticle: This is the hard bit of skin that lines the edges of your finger and toenails.

Essential Oil: This is a very pure form of a plant, herb, or flower. When diluted and added to lotion or water, essential oils can be very soothing, but they can really pack a punch ... so be sure to mix essential oils with something else before applying them directly to your skin!

Exfoliate: OK, it sounds creepy but your body sheds dry (or dead) skin cells – constantly. Yup, constantly. Using a body or face scrub can help your body exfoliate (or get rid of) that yucky-old dead skin. After a nice gentle scrub, your "new" skin will glow just like a baby's .

Facial: A facial is a luxurious way to improve the skin on your face (a.k.a. your complexion). It can help deep clean, moisturize, balance, or do whatever your skin needs to be perfect and pimple-free. Plus, it feels amazing!

Manicure: A manicure is a deluxe treatment for your hands and fingernails. It can include massage, pushing back cuticles, and filing and polishing the nails.

Massage: Like to be pampered? A massage is one of the most relaxing spa treatments available. It's good for the mind, body, and soul! If you've never had one, it can take some getting used to. It involves rubbing or kneading your muscles. It's usually performed on the back, but is great for the legs, feet, arms, and hands, too!

Moisturize: This is VERY important. After cleansing and toning your face or body, applying a nice moisturizer will help your skin stay soft, supple, and young.

Pedicure: Just like a manicure, only for your toes! Some girls consider it a necessity, especially in the summertime. A pedicure usually includes a foot scrub, massage, cuticle removal, and (of course) a polish.

Pumice Stone: This is a light piece of rock used to rub away those dead, hard bits of skin on your feet.

Steam: Steam can be annoying when it fogs up the mirror after a nice hot shower, but it's great for your skin. It's an excellent way to open your pores, which are those little tiny holes in your skin that help your good-old epidermis breathe. Gyms and spas have special steam rooms that help you relax and get you glowing.

Toner: Toner is a basic step in your facial cleansing routine. It's a light liquid that removes all traces of dirt on the face. It also closes the pores and prepares the face for a moisturizer.

For Good Measure

You don't have to be too persnickety when measuring out ingredients for your recipes, but it's important to get your ratios at least pretty close to correct. Use the back edge of a butter knife to level off the ingredients in your spoon or cup and remember to wash utensils with soap and water after each use. When a recipe calls for a "drop" of something, use an eye-dropper (and squeeze slowly!). Luckily, many essential oils come with tops that release just one drop at a time. If you like one scent more than another in the recipe, get creative and add an extra drop of your favorite (and one less of the other) oil into the mixture. Also, for sanitation's sake, be sure to wash eye-droppers with hot soapy water.

Stocking Up AND Staying Safe

You could do major damage to your piggy bank by stocking up on the latest beauty products. There are way too many must-haves to keep up with. But looking your best doesn't have to mean killing your college savings – you CAN recreate many treatments at home with just a few common ingredients and a little in*spa*ration!

Things you'll need:

Carrier oils: Any oil that's labeled "extra virgin" or "cold-pressed" will work as a carrier. Sweet almond, grapeseed, canola, and olive oil are all easy to find at grocery, drug, or health food stores.

Essential oils: There's a scent out there for every mood. Lavender, lemon, and peppermint oil are popular and smell great. You can find your favorite at just about any good health food store or drugstore.

Fruits and veggies: Bananas, papayas, cucumbers, and avocados are not just yummy to eat – they're a soothing treat for your skin!

Honey: A sweet benefit for the hair and skin.

Oatmeal: Great for delicate body scrubs and face masks.

Dried lavender: One of the most soothing scents you can sniff! Lavender is sooooo relaxing that it'll actually help you snooze better. You can buy a bag or jar of it at quality craft stores and gourmet grocery stores.

Sea salt or kosher salt: This stuff is chunkier than normal table salt. Ask for it at grocery, health, or gourmet food stores.

Distilled water: This is special purified water. You can find it at the grocery store or drugstore.

Glass or stainless steel bowls in different sizes: Check out your kitchen cupboards or go to any housewares shop.

Measuring cups and spoons: Borrow from your parents or buy a nice inexpensive set from the grocery store.

Safety scissors: You'll need to keep all your fingers for those deluxe manicures, so we suggest investing in a special pair of safety scissors. You can find them at most stationery, fabric, or drugstores.

Lotion/moisturizer: There are SO many types of good quality moisturizers on the market. Get whatever suits you best (i.e. sensitive, dry, or oily skin). Don't skimp!

Hand towels, bath towels, and washcloths: Raid the linen closet. (But ask for permission first!)

Mood music: Mellow, peppy, sophisticated – it's really up to you. Ask friends to bring their favorite sounds.

Safety First!

Cooking and baking can be loads of fun, but they can also be dangerous. (They don't call those bits on the stovetop "burners" for nothing!) So be sure to get permission from your parents or guardian before throwing on that cute apron and raiding the kitchen cupboards. And, most importantly, ALWAYS ask an adult to supervise when you need to use the oven or stove.

Feeling Testy?

When it comes to beauty treatments, taking a test is actually a good thing! Your skin may be sensitive to certain ingredients and it would be a major pain to break out in a rash. Dab a little sample of any lotion, oils, masks, etc. on the inside of your wrist before slathering anything on your face or body. This is called a "patch test." Wait an hour or so to see if you have any sort of allergic reaction. If you notice redness, bumps, or blotchiness, DON'T use the treatment.

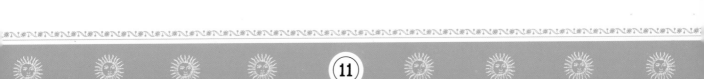

SPAGHETTI

Have fun with food! Besides feeding your inside, edibles can be great for your outside. Common fruits and vegetables can clean and soothe your face, hair, and body. And they smell fabulous, too! So, make a grocery list, shop till you drop, and invite over a few friends.

First, get the ambience right by placing colorful fruits and veggies in bowls around the kitchen. Think cucumbers, carrots, apples, oranges, and red (or yellow) peppers. Throw a bright plastic-coated tablecloth over the kitchen counter (or wherever your work space is) to catch any spills. And make sure you don't have the munchies before you start – you'll need all the goodies you've got to get glam. Lastly, tie on a stylish apron and start cookin'!

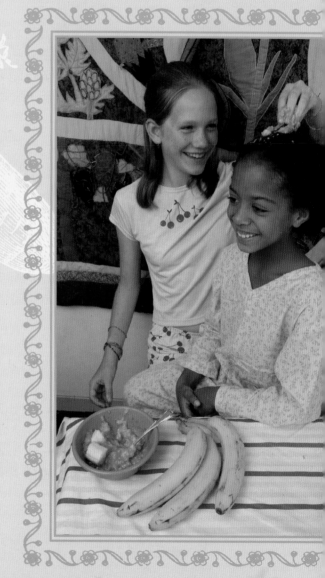

SAUCY SPAGHETTI

This zesty fresh tomato and basil *Spa*ghetti is an ideal snack for your kitchen crew.

3 tablespoons olive oil
1 clove garlic, minced
2 14-ounce cans diced tomatoes
1/4 teaspoon salt

1/4 teaspoon black pepper
8-ounces dried spaghetti
10-15 basil leaves
Grated Parmesan cheese

Pour the oil into a large sauté pan on the stove and turn the heat to low. Add the minced garlic. Give the garlic a stir and wait for it to start sizzling (and smelling good!). In the meantime, open the cans of tomatoes. Once the garlic is sizzling (and just beginning to turn golden), carefully add the tomatoes and stir. Turn the heat to high until the sauce boils, then turn it back to low. Stir the sauce every few minutes. It should take about 20 minutes for the sauce to thicken. While the sauce is cooking, fill a big pot with water and put a lid on it. Ask an adult to help you put it on the stove and turn the heat to high. After the water starts to boil, remove the lid using a potholder. Carefully drop the spaghetti into the boiling water. Stir the pasta so it doesn't stick together. Let it cook for seven minutes. Don't forget to stir the sauce! Ask an adult to help you drain the pasta and pour some oil over it while it's still warm so it doesn't stick together. To finish the sauce, stack the basil leaves on top of each other. Carefully trim the basil into small pieces (with kitchen scissors) right into the sauce. Add salt and pepper … and stir! Divide the pasta into four bowls and ladle the sauce over the pasta. Sprinkle with Parmesan cheese and serve.

Makes four servings.

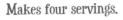

Spa Specialities

SPA EATS

SAUCY SPAGHETTI

SPA TREATS

GO BANANAS HAIR TREATMENT

FUNNY HONEY MOISTURE MASK

TEA BAG TONER AND EYE SOOTHER

SPA SUPPLIES

1 ripe banana
Plastic wrap

Go Bananas Hair Treatment

Bananas are much more than monkey food – they're a naturally awesome way to moisturize your skin and hair.

Shampoo and towel dry hair. ◎ Peel the banana and mash it with a fork in a small bowl. ◎ Scoop up the banana mash with your fingers and run it through your hair, as though you were applying a thick conditioner. ◎ Wrap your hair in plastic wrap. Lie back and relax (in silky pjs and fuzzy slippers – or whatever suits your mood) for 15 minutes and let the banana work its magic. ◎ Next, rinse thoroughly with warm water and let your hair air-dry. ◎ Enjoy your silky locks all day long. For ultimate pampering, apply the Funny Honey Moisture Mask and Tea Bag Eye Soother at the same time.

SPA SUPPLIES

2 teaspoons pure honey
1 teaspoon oatmeal
(optional)

Funny Honey Moisture Mask

To soothe irritated, flaky skin, mix a spoonful of oatmeal into some honey and then gently rub it on your face.

Pure honey is a mega-moisturizer! If your skin is dry (which happens a lot in the winter), spread a thick layer of gooey goodness over your face, avoiding your eyes. ◎ Unwind for 15 minutes and wash off with warm water. ◎ Gently towel dry your face and voilà … you've got smooth, soft (and sweet!) cheeks.

Tea Bag Toner and Eye Soother

For a finishing touch, toner is a great way to have super-clean skin. It feels tingly and good, too!

SPA SUPPLIES

2 chamomile tea bags
Cotton balls

Making your own toner sounds technical, but it's actually as easy as making a cup of tea. Steep two tea bags in a cup of hot tap water for about five minutes. ☺ Put the cup (with the tea bags still in it) in the refrigerator for one full hour. ☺ Put on some nice music, relax, and gab with your girlfriends while you wait. ☺ Take the chilled tea out of the fridge, dip a cotton ball into the cup, and delicately rub it all over your face. Let your skin dry naturally.

☺ But wait! You're not done indulging just yet. Tea bags help reduce puffiness and dark circles. ☺ Take the tea bags out of the cup and lightly squeeze them to remove excess liquid. ☺ Place one over each eyelid, lean back, and luxuriate. ☺ Toss the bags once you feel fully relaxed and fabulous.

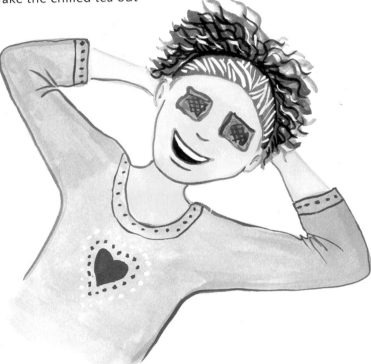

WISH UPON A SPA

Make your next slumber *spa*rty a night to remember! Instead of telling scary stories that will give you nightmares, make wishes. If it's too cloudy to wish upon a star, don't worry – munch on a Star Wish Cookie instead. Or you could chill out by breathing in some lovely lavender and rosemary. And when you are pooped from too much partying, climb into your sleeping bag and curl up with your dream pouch. That way, you and your friends are sure to have sweet dreams all night long.

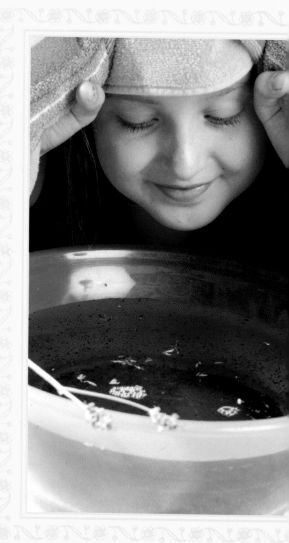

STAR WISH COOKIES

Wish upon a star when you make these star-shaped sugar cookies.

1 cup all-purpose flour
1/4 teaspoon salt
1/4 teaspoon baking powder
4 tablespoons butter, softened
1/2 cup granulated sugar
1 egg
1/2 teaspoon vanilla extract
Star-shaped cookie cutter, optional

In a medium bowl, sift the flour, salt, and baking powder together and set aside. In a large bowl, cream the butter and sugar with a wooden spoon or hand mixer. Beat in the egg and vanilla extract. Add the flour mixture to the butter and sugar mixture and stir until blended. Place the dough on a sheet of waxed paper. Use the palm of your hand to form the dough into a square about 1-inch thick. Wrap and refrigerate for 30 minutes. Preheat the oven to 400 degrees. On a floured work surface, roll the dough to about 1/4-inch thick. Add more flour as needed to keep the dough from sticking. Use the cookie cutter or a dull knife to cut the dough into star shapes or any shape you like. Place the cut cookies on a cookie sheet using a wide spatula. Re-roll the dough scraps and cut again into more cookies. Ask an adult to help you put the cookie sheet in the oven. Bake the cookies for 8-10 minutes. Remove the cookie sheet from the oven with potholders. Using a spatula, transfer the cookies to a wire rack to cool.

Makes about 16 cookies.

Spa Specialities

SPA EATS

STAR WISH COOKIES

SPA TREATS

DREAM POUCH

LAVENDER-ROSEMARY FACIAL STEAM DREAMS

     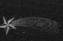 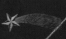

SPA SUPPLIES

1 teaspoon dried
  rosemary
1 teaspoon dried lavender

Lavender-Rosemary Facial Steam Dreams

For centuries, people have used herbs to have sweet dreams and restful sleep. But rosemary and lavender also have added beauty benefits: rosemary perks up your skin; lavender calms and soothes. So treat yourself to an herbal facial steam before bed for a good night's sleep and a healthy glow!

Fill up your bathroom sink (or a large bowl) with warm tap water. Sprinkle the herbs into the water and cover the sink with a bath towel for several minutes. This will help the herbs to steep in the water (just like when you're making tea). Now, pull back your hair and lean your face 6-12 inches above the water. Drape the towel over your head (like a tent). Breathe in deeply and allow the steam to open your pores. Relax in this position for about 10 minutes. Do you feel your skin tingling? Rinse your face with cool water – and don't forget to clean up the sink or basin before you head to bed!

Dream Pouch

Some people believe that slipping a wish inside a small pillow can help make dreams come true. Now you can take control of your destiny and make your very own dream pouch in just a couple of minutes!

Lay fabric on a desk or table. Place a tablespoon (or two) of rice in the center of the fabric. Write your wish on a small slip of paper. Roll the paper into a small scroll and place it on top of the rice. Gather up each edge of the fabric and tie a pretty string (or cord) around the top of your pouch. Be sure to knot it tightly so no rice falls out during the night. Place the pouch under your pillow ... and prepare to have your wish come true!

Power SPA

You've probably heard the ads that say milk "does a body good." But there are lots of other ways to build strong bones and relax your muscles. Make a tasty yogurt *Spar*fait and invite a few friends over for a super soothing massage. Massage (or bodywork) is one of the best – and most beneficial – spa treats. Some say the Chinese developed it thousands of years ago and many experts believe it's a powerful healer of both the mind and the body. Professionals (a.k.a. massage therapists) go to school to learn this ancient art and perfect their techniques, of which there are lots of different types: Swedish, Stone, Shiatsu and Deep Tissue – just to name a few! With some warm stones and yummy body butter, you can give your friends a backrub they'll never forget, even though you're not a pro.

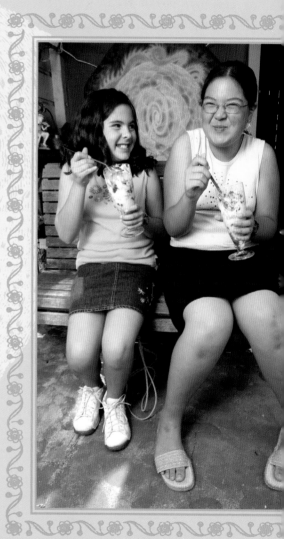

YOGURT SPARFAIT

Yogurt doesn't just taste good – all that calcium is good for you, right down to the bone! So treat your body right with this tasty parfait.

1 8-ounce package of vanilla yogurt
1 pint of raspberries
1-2 cups granola

Place serving glasses on the counter next to the ingredients. ❦ Put one heaping tablespoon of granola in the bottom of the cups. ❦ Put one heaping tablespoon of yogurt on top of the granola and spread it to the edges of the cup. ❦ Put a layer of raspberries on top of the yogurt. ❦ Now start all over again, repeating the layers of granola, yogurt, and fruit. ❦ Finish with a final layer of yogurt.

*Also, try peaches with strawberry yogurt or strawberries with maple yogurt for variety!

Makes two servings.

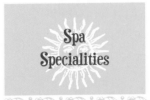

Spa Specialities

SPA EATS

YOGURT SPARFAIT

SPA TREATS

WARM STONE MASSAGE

BODY BUTTER

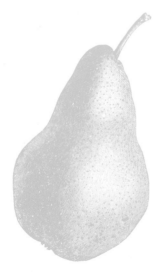

SPA SUPPLIES

6 large stones

Warm Stone Massage

Smooth flat rocks work best for this relaxing treat. You should be able to find lots of good ones by a pond, river, lake, or ocean. Once you collect your stones, take them home and give 'em a good scrub with hot soapy water. Place all your stones in a sink (or a large bowl) filled with hot (but not scalding) tap water. Let the stones heat up until they feel warm to the touch (about 10 minutes). You may need to add more hot water after the first five minutes, to keep the temperature warm enough. ◎ Put on some mellow music and you're ready to give a super-duper relaxing rub down! Have whoever's first throw on a bikini and lay face down on a flat comfy surface. Place the warm stones next to the lucky girl and instruct her to breathe deeply. Start by gently massaging her shoulders and applying pressure with your thumbs and palms. After a few minutes of massage, lay a warm stone on one of her shoulders. Let the stone rest there for several minutes so the stone's heat penetrates to the muscle. Repeat on the other shoulder with a new rock. ◎ Continue this method as you work your way down her back and spine, massaging each area first with your fingers and palms, and then laying a warm stone on the muscle.

Body Butter

Stiff from carrying too many textbooks and lugging around that big fat backpack? Watch your friend's muscles melt with pleasure – and help beautify her back at the same time – with this divine body butter treatment. It not only smells delicious, but the eucalyptus oil will soothe those aching muscles.

Making it is simple: just peel and mash the banana and avocado together in one bowl (you can use your hands or a potato masher). Try to get the ingredients as smooth as possible! Add 1 drop of eucalyptus oil and mix. ◎ Place a bath towel on a flat surface, have your friend put on a bikini top and lie face down. Smooth the body butter over your friend's back and have her relax on her stomach for about 10 or 15 minutes. She can cap her treatment by rinsing in a nice warm shower. Yum!

SPA SUPPLIES

- 1 ripe banana
- 1 ripe avocado
- 1 drop eucalyptus essential oil
- 1 bowl
- 1 bath towel

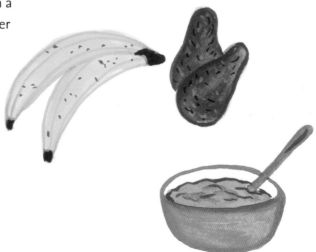

MA AND SPA

If you stopped to think about it, you'd realize that your mom has devoted a lot of time over the years waiting on you hand and foot. Now it's your turn to treat her like a queen for the day! Give her a hand with a magnificent "momicure." Treat her to a fruity facial and help her face the world with bright eyes and beautiful skin. Then, when you're finished with the pampering, spend some mother-daughter bonding time by baking (and breaking) bread together.

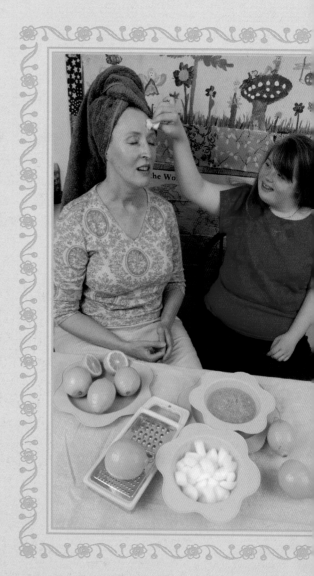

WELL-BRED BANANA BREAD

Bake a loaf of bread that even grandma would be proud of!

3 ripe bananas
2 eggs, beaten
2 cups flour
3/4 cup sugar
1 teaspoon salt
1 1/2 teaspoons baking soda
1/2 cup walnuts, chopped

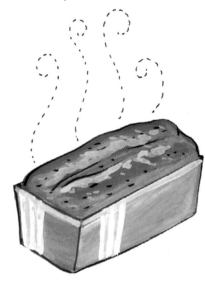

Preheat oven to 350 degrees and spray an 8 1/2 x 4 1/2 x 3-inch loaf pan with nonstick cooking spray. 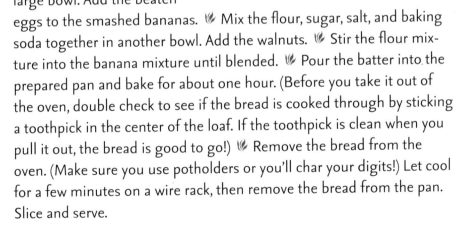 Peel the bananas and smash them in a large bowl. Add the beaten eggs to the smashed bananas. Mix the flour, sugar, salt, and baking soda together in another bowl. Add the walnuts. Stir the flour mixture into the banana mixture until blended. Pour the batter into the prepared pan and bake for about one hour. (Before you take it out of the oven, double check to see if the bread is cooked through by sticking a toothpick in the center of the loaf. If the toothpick is clean when you pull it out, the bread is good to go!) Remove the bread from the oven. (Make sure you use potholders or you'll char your digits!) Let cool for a few minutes on a wire rack, then remove the bread from the pan. Slice and serve.

Makes one loaf and serves four to six.

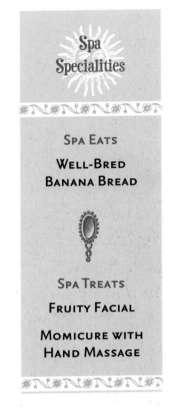

SPA Specialities

SPA EATS
WELL-BRED BANANA BREAD

SPA TREATS
FRUITY FACIAL

MOMICURE WITH HAND MASSAGE

SPA SUPPLIES

2 lemons

Favorite face moisturizer

Fruity Facial

Citrus fruits (like lemons and oranges) have natural acids that can help cure dry, flaky skin.

Squeeze the juice out of two lemons and grate the rind (or peel) of the fruit. Place the juice and the rind in a bowl and cover it with plastic wrap. Let the mixture chill in the fridge overnight. Once the mixture is chilled and ready to go, pull mom's hair back from her face and fasten with a clip or rubber band. Pat the mixture over her face (make sure she's makeup free first!). Have mom kick back and relax for a few minutes while the mix dries and then gently wash it off with a warm washcloth. Smooth on a few drops of her favorite moisturizer to complete the facial. Now have mom try some on you. You'll both be glowing in no time!

Momicure with Hand Massage

Fill a small bowl with soapy water and place your mom's fingertips in it. After a few minutes, remove one hand. ◎ Shape each nail with a nail file (file straight across and slightly round on the edges). Using a quarter-sized dollop of lotion, massage her hand. ◎ With your thumb on her palm and fingers on the back of her hand, gently press and massage between each finger. Pay special attention to the fleshy area between the thumb and index finger. Press and hold each fingertip for several seconds and release. Use your thumb to press and stroke her wrist and palm. ◎ Continue massaging her hand until the lotion is absorbed into the skin. ◎ Remove her other hand from the soapy water and repeat the process. ◎ After you've finished massaging both hands, dip a cotton ball in nail polish remover and wipe each fingernail clean. ◎ Carefully apply a base coat of clear nail polish to each finger and let dry for two minutes. Apply your mom's color of choice to each nail. Top with a coat of clear polish and let air-dry for 10-20 minutes.

While mom's fingernails are busy drying, do her toes!

SPA SUPPLIES

Liquid soap
Nail file
Hand lotion
Cotton balls
Nail polish remover
Clear nail polish
Favorite nail polish

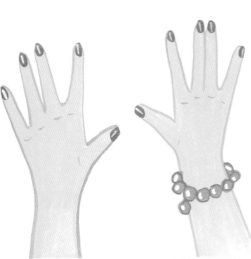

Pooches and pussycats like pampering, too! They give you love every day so return the favor with this ultimate pet spa. Invite your friends and tell them to bring their pets with them. Make sure a litter box is available for the kitties and put down paper if there are untrained puppies in attendance. Put bowls of dog biscuits and cat treats around the room and open your pet spa. Spritz the dogs with Pooch Potion and massage the cats to pet nirvana. One note of caution: Your pet may never want to go to the groomer again!

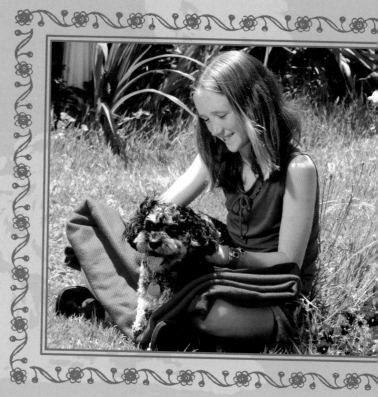

CREATURE COOKIES

Make sure your pets don't go hungry!

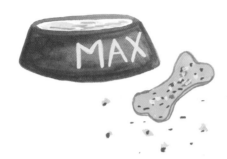

2 cups whole-wheat flour

1/2 cup corn meal

1/2 teaspoon salt

2 2 1/2-ounce jars of beef,
   chicken, or lamb baby food

2 eggs

1/3 cup milk

1/4 cup cooking oil

Preheat the oven to 350 degrees. ❧ In a large bowl, mix the flour, corn meal, and salt. ❧ In another bowl whisk together the baby food, eggs, milk, and oil. ❧ Add the baby food mix to the flour mix and stir until blended. ❧ On a floured work surface, roll the dough to about 1/4-inch thick. Add more flour as needed to keep the dough from sticking. ❧ Using a dull knife, cut the dough into tantalizing creature shapes like dog bones or triangle-shaped wedges of cheese. Remember: small pets need small critter cookies. ❧ Using a wide spatula, transfer the cookies to a cookie sheet. ❧ Bake the cookies for 25-30 minutes. ❧ Remove the cookie sheet from the oven and put it on a cooling rack. Wait for the Creature Cookies to cool before serving them to your pooch or kitty.

Spa Specialities

SPA EATS
CREATURE COOKIES

SPA TREATS
POOCH POTION

PET MASSAGE

SPA SUPPLIES

2 cups water
1 tea bag (chamomile or peppermint)
1 tablespoon of cider vinegar
Metal bowl

Pooch Potion

Make a stink-busting treat for your dog with this vinegar-based shampoo. (Like baking soda, vinegar is a potent odor-eater.) This spray is the perfect thing to mist on your dog's coat while you are brushing him or her. It's so light that it won't bother your pooch's sensitive nose. Both you and your pet will appreciate his/her fresh, clean coat!

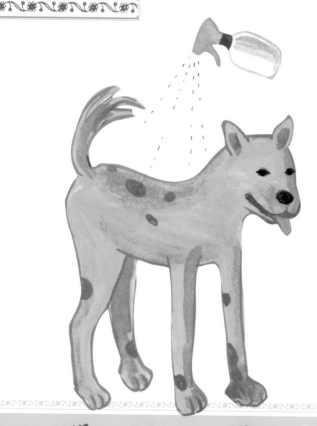

To get started, boil two cups of water. ◎ Pour the heated water over the tea bag of your choice into a metal bowl. ◎ Cover the bowl and let steep. ◎ After about 15 minutes, put the tea in the refrigerator for 1 hour. ◎ Once it is cold, add vinegar and put the potion in a spray bottle. ◎ In your best snazzy writing, date and label the bottle "Pooch Potion." ◎ Refrigerate leftover spray for next time.

Pet Massage

Your pets will love you even more after you rub them down! Many trained professionals believe that massage has the same healing benefits for pets as it does for humans. You can actually take classes or buy videos on proper technique! If you haven't massaged or rubbed your pet before, be careful. Don't hold your pet down if he/she doesn't want to lie still. Be gentle and make the massage into a game. If they think you want to play, they'll play along!

Use your palms for big dogs. Use your fingers for cats and small dogs. Gently rub in small circular motions. 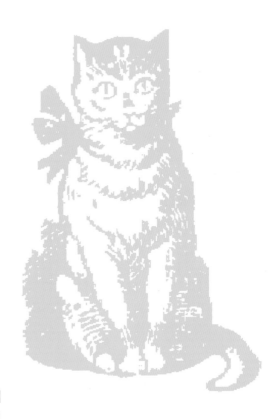 Start with the feet and paws. Move up the leg. If your pet is enjoying the massage, move onto his/her stomach. Your pet may even roll onto his/her back so you have easier access. Cats may not like their stomachs rubbed. If he/she doesn't like it, ignore this area and move onto the back. Massage the neck, head, and ears. If your pet likes what you are doing, don't stop! Spend time stroking the ears from base to tip, or gently rub them between your index finger and thumb. Don't forget the tail!

Solar SPA

Ever notice that being outside on a sunny day can actually make you feel happier? It's time to take charge and pull back your curtains, or (even better) get your booty in gear and get yourself outside. In ancient Egypt, people worshipped the sun god, Ra. Now you can host a deluxe outdoor *spa*rty and do your own modern-day sun worshipping in style. Feel the warmth, soak up the rays, and try a fun yoga move we call a Sun *Spa*lutation. Be sure to wear your most comfortable sweats and plenty of sunscreen. Afterwards, take a moment to lie back on the grass and stare at the clouds. Consider it daydreaming, just kicking back, or meditating – whatever works! Either way, you'll be toasty and relaxed.

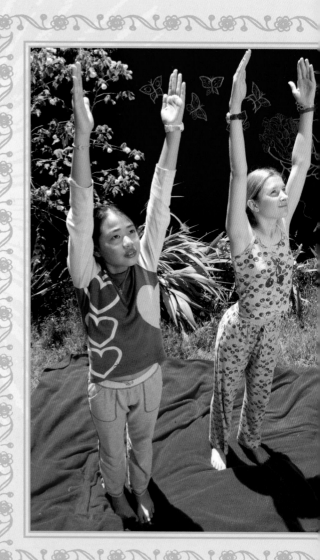

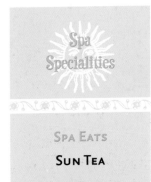

SUN TEA

Sun tea is an American invention that brews – just as the name suggests – in the heat of the sun.

8 cups cold water
8 bags of black tea
Extra water or ice (if desired)

8-16 teaspoons granulated sugar
Ice cubes

Combine water and tea bags in a pitcher or glass bowl.  Cover the top with plastic wrap (so no critters will get in). Set it outside in the sun and let the tea bags steep for at least three hours. Dilute with water or ice to get the color (and taste) you prefer. If the tea looks and tastes too weak for your liking, add more tea bags and wait a little longer for the sun to do its magic. Stir in one or two teaspoons of sugar for each cup of tea just before serving. Serve this yummy all-natural concoction over ice in a nice tall glass, sit back, and drink up the sun!

Makes about a dozen large glasses.

SOLAR ENERGY SNACK

Have fun in the sun and munch on a simple sunflower trail mix.

2 cups sunflower seeds
1/2 cup raisins
1/2 cup chocolate chips
1/2 cup peanuts
1/2 cup mini-pretzels

1/2 cup of any of these optional ingredients: grated coconut, M&M's, walnuts, cashews, dried apricots – or anything you think sounds good!

Toss all the ingredients together in a pretty bowl. Gather friends, grab some sun tea, serve, and enjoy.

Makes four servings.

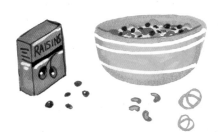

Eye on the Sky

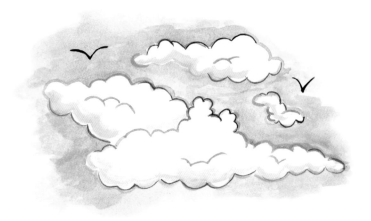

Face it: life can be pretty hectic sometimes. It's important to take a little time each and every day for yourself to chill out, unwind, and take a mental break. Meditation is a great way to liberate yourself from everyday stressors like school, friends, homework, crushes, chores, and everything else you've got going on. When you meditate, you empty the mind or focus your thoughts on just one thing. It's takes some getting used to, but once you master it, meditation can help improve your concentration and make you feel totally renewed.

One of the keys to meditation is to free your mind. Another is to find something to focus on. It sounds silly, but simply staring into space is a great way to do both of these. Try looking at clouds in the sky. To get started, head outside, find a nice patch of grass in a private place, and lie down. If it's a sunny day, make sure you wear shades and don't look directly at the sun! Every time a thought comes into your head, acknowledge it but let go of it immediately. The more you focus on the clouds, the more you will forget all your worries!

Sun *Spa*lutations

These days, doing yoga is almost as popular as wearing tanks or watching reality TV. But yoga has been healing minds and bodies for centuries. Created in India, it's an age-old practice of breathing exercises and body postures. People who study yoga feel calmer, healthier, and are more flexible. Start your day with a few of what we call Sun *Spa*lutations (a basic sequence of movements) and let yoga work its magic on you. You'll be amazed at how great you'll look and feel after a yoga workout.

The original sun salutation is a series of "asanas" (the yoga term for "pose" or "position") that warms you up and makes you strong and flexible. Focus on your breathing. Put a hand on your chest and feel your breath going in and out of your lungs. ☺ Begin by standing with your feet hip-width apart. Your hands should hang by your sides. As you breathe in, bring your arms up overhead. Arch your back and look up. As you breath out, bend over and try to touch your toes. Bend your knees if you can't reach the floor. Then breathe in and bring your body up slowly with your arms out to the sides. Bring arms over your head and look up. Breathe out, slowly lowering your arms to your sides. End by bringing your palms together in front of your chest. This is called the "prayer position." ☺ Repeat this sequence several times and you're sure to feel sunny on the inside and out!

Ah SPA!

Feeling yucky, icky, clammy, and not so hot? You may not know it, but there are tons of therapeutic tricks stocked in your very own kitchen cupboard and bathroom cabinet. Ever heard that gargling with salt water can help cure a sore throat? How about that a spoonful of sugar can stop hiccups? Sure, some so-called homemade medical miracles are just old wives' tales, but almost everyone has at least one home remedy that he/she swears by. Share yours with friends and treat yourselves to the very best in home tonics – a warm bath, a soothing rub, and some tasty chicken soup. Aches, pains, and homework be gone … if only for a day!

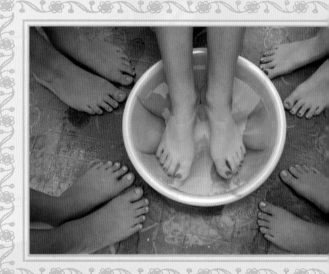

KICKIN' CHICKEN SOUP

Kick any aches and pains, chills or ills with a good old-fashioned cure-all: a cup of chicken soup.

2 tablespoons vegetable oil
1/2 cup finely sliced onion
1/2 cup finely sliced carrot
1/4 cup finely sliced celery
1 cup cooked chicken meat,
    cut into cubes
1 14-ounce can of chicken broth
2 cups water
1 cup fine egg noodles
1 tablespoon chopped parsley

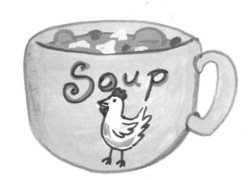

Pour the oil into a medium-sized soup pan and turn the heat on the stove to medium. 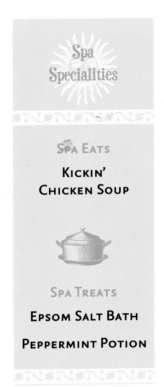 Add the onion, carrot, and celery and cook for three to four minutes (or until the onions are soft and golden). Add the chicken, chicken broth, and water. Turn the heat to high and bring the broth to a boil. When the broth boils, turn the heat to low and add the noodles. Stir the soup and let it cook for five minutes more. Turn off the heat. Sprinkle the parsley over the soup and carefully ladle each serving into a nice big bowl or cup.

Makes four servings.

Spa
Specialities

SPA EATS

KICKIN'
CHICKEN SOUP

SPA TREATS

EPSOM SALT BATH

PEPPERMINT POTION

SPA SUPPLIES

1 cup Epsom salt
1 tablespoon baby oil

Epsom Salt Bath

People have been using Epsom salt to soothe their spirits for a long, long time. This special salt is named for the mineral-rich waters of Epsom, England and is known to have miraculous medicinal benefits. Try soaking your tootsies to relieve aches, remove odors, and soften skin. Or just sink your whole body into a good old-fashioned therapeutic bath and feel your cares float away!

Add the salt and oil to your bath or bowl and let the healing qualities of the salt do its work.

Epsom: Seriously Super Salt!

- Rub a handful on wet skin and it'll cleanse, exfoliate, and soften rough spots.

- Gently press a warm salt-soaked compress on insect bites to take the sting out.

- Press a cold salt-soaked compress on a sprain or bruise to reduce swelling

- Get an extra-fresh face by mixing half a teaspoonful into your regular cleanser.

- Soak your finger in a mix of salt and warm water to draw out a nasty splinter.

- Add bounce and volume to your hair by combining equal parts of conditioner and salt. (Then just warm the mixture in a pan, work it into hair, let sit for 20 minutes, rinse, and go!)

- Feed some to your plants to keep them happy and healthy.

Peppermint Potion

This zesty oil will clear your head and lift your ailing spirits!

Mix the essential oils with the sweet almond oil or any other carrier oil. (You can use grapeseed oil, jojoba oil, or even canola oil from the kitchen as your carrier.) ◎ Place a few drops of the mixture on your fingertips and rub your friend's temples. (The temples are located a couple of inches above the ears, right at the hairline.) ◎ Have your friend relax and take deep breaths to clear her head. ◎ Once you've done the temples, take a few more drops of potion and begin rubbing her neck and shoulders. ◎ Use your thumbs to apply gentle pressure to the back of her neck and rub in small circles. She'll feel divine in no time!

Remember, essential oils are very potent concentrations of flowers and herbs. You should never put these oils directly on the skin. They need to be mixed with something else to be used safely.

SPA SUPPLIES

- 2 drops lavender essential oil
- 2 drops peppermint essential oil
- 2 drops rosemary essential oil
- 2 tablespoons sweet almond oil

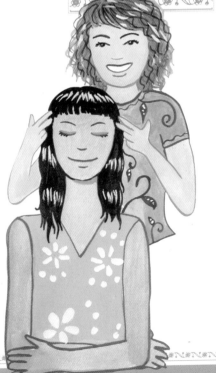

  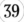

SPA FROM AFAR

People all over the world have their own ways to unwind. In India young women meditate. In Finland, they enjoy a sauna to soothe tired muscles. In Japan, they walk in mazes and giant Zen gardens to unwind. Fortunately, you don't have to be a globe-trotter to enjoy a few of these exotic treats from afar – you can actually do it all in your own bedroom and backyard! Learn the ancient art of Tai Chi or create a magical Zen garden that will calm and entertain you long after the *spa*rty's over.

Set the right mood by bringing out souvenirs from far-off places. Wear colorful clothing or a T-shirt from your favorite vacation location. Let your imagination travel far and wide!

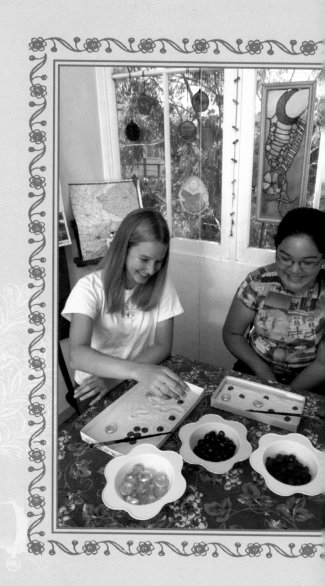

SLOTH BROTH

Start your day of Zen relaxation with a comforting bowl of noodle soup.

2 14-ounce cans of chicken or
     vegetable broth
2 cups water
3 ounces dried ramen noodles
1/2 cup frozen peas
1 cup firm tofu or cooked chicken,
     cut into small cubes
1/4 cup green onions, trimmed and
     cut into small circles
1/2 teaspoon soy sauce

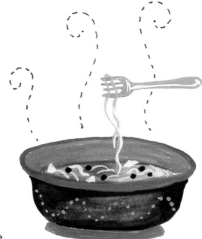

Pour the broth and the water into a
medium soup pan and turn the stove
to medium heat. 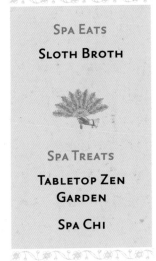 When the broth boils,
turn the heat to low, add the noodles, and simmer for five minutes.
 Add the peas, tofu, and green onions and simmer for two more
minutes. Turn off the heat and stir in the soy sauce. Carefully
ladle into bowls and serve.

Makes four servings.

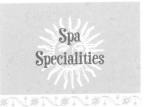

SPA SUPPLIES

1 cup sand (or salt)
4-6 small pebbles
Shoebox lid
Toothpick, fork,
   or chopstick

Tabletop Zen Garden

If yardwork sounds more like a chore than a soul soother, you've never experienced the art of a Japanese Zen garden. Some Zen gardens are as big (or bigger) than a real-life traditional garden, but you can make a mini version and enjoy the same benefits.

Pour a cup of sand into the upside-down shoebox lid. Artfully place the pebbles in whatever pattern you wish. Use a toothpick, fork, or chopstick to create cool designs in the sand. If you want to change your garden, just gently shake from side to side and start over!

Now and Zen

Zen gardens aren't as simple as they look. There's a whole philosophy and history behind them, dating back to ancient monasteries in Japan. If you've ever seen one, you'll notice just two main elements: rocks and sand.

Zen gardeners use rocks to make mini mountains (or islands) and sand to symbolize flowing water. In Japan, islands are a symbol of longevity and lasting health. Most Zen gardens have single and multiple rock island formations. Sometimes the islands are

built to resemble the shape of a tortoise or a crane (a type of tall, wading bird). Both animals represent long life. The tortoise is believed to live for 10,000 years and the crane for 1,000 years!

Bridges are also common in Zen gardens. They allow people a path to cross the "seas" and connect islands to one another. They also open up a new view that might not have been noticed from below. Pretty cool, huh?

  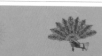

Spa Chi

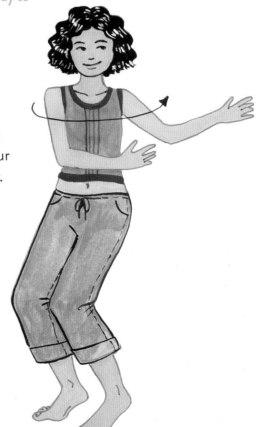

Tai Chi (TY-CHEE) may look easy (and a little goofy), but it's good for your body – and your soul. According to historians, Tai Chi began many centuries ago in China as a way for warriors to stay physically fit as they grew older. Try this simple variation called Spa Chi for a unique way to relax indoors and out.

Find a quiet place. Start with your feet about a foot apart. Your hands should be relaxed (but not limp). Keep your back straight and bend your knees slightly. ◎ Move your arms and hands in slow, flowing movements. Your eyes should follow your hands. ◎ Think of the upper body as a corkscrew. Turn right or left from the waist only. Do not bend forward or backward. Do not turn your head from side to side; it should only move with your upper body. ◎ Keep your feet rooted to the ground. Try to repeat a sequence of arm movements after a few minutes.

If you want, pick a leader to stand in front of the rest of the group. Try to follow her movements out of the corner of your eye. And no giggling! Just relax and continue to focus on your own hands and arms.

 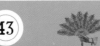

SENSE-SATIONAL SPA

It's time to come to your senses and follow your nose! Aromatherapy uses different smells to affect our moods. Some smells, like peppermint, help give us energy. Others, like lavender, help send us to sleep. And some smells, like vanilla, can even make us hungry!

Sounds can also have a big impact on how we feel. Good music can make your spirits soar, while the sound of waves gently crashing on a beach can help you catch some snooze time. The soft sounds of the wind through the trees or chimes can soothe your soul and lift your spirit.

So get creative and invite your friends over for a sense-sational day!

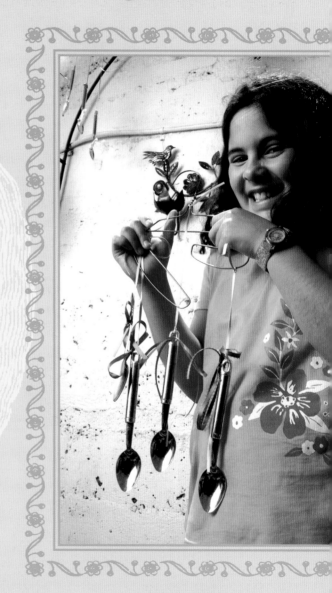

HEAVEN-SCENT CINNAMON CRISP

Nothing smells better than cinnamon baking, so soothe your senses with this sweet treat.

3 cups peaches (fresh, frozen, or canned) or any combination of
   peaches, raspberries, blueberries, or strawberries
1/4 cup sugar
1/4 cup brown sugar
1 cup all-purpose flour
1 teaspoon cinnamon
1/4 teaspoon powdered ginger
1/2 teaspoon salt
1 stick (or 1/2 cup) of cold butter, cut into
   small cubes
Vanilla ice cream

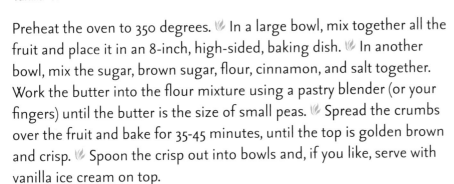

Preheat the oven to 350 degrees. In a large bowl, mix together all the fruit and place it in an 8-inch, high-sided, baking dish. In another bowl, mix the sugar, brown sugar, flour, cinnamon, and salt together. Work the butter into the flour mixture using a pastry blender (or your fingers) until the butter is the size of small peas. Spread the crumbs over the fruit and bake for 35-45 minutes, until the top is golden brown and crisp. Spoon the crisp out into bowls and, if you like, serve with vanilla ice cream on top.

Makes six servings.

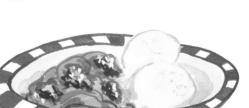

Spa Specialities

SPA EATS

HEAVEN-SCENT CINNAMON CRISP

SPA TREATS

CHARMING CHIMES

ROCKIN' ROOM FRESHENER

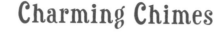

SPA SUPPLIES

Old keys
Spoons and forks
Other found items
Thick string or cord
Glue
Metal coat hanger

Charming Chimes

Stir your soul with the tinkling music of wind chimes. Gather your materials together. (All you need is a bunch of stuff from the junk drawer!) ☺ Cut a piece of string for each item you have. ☺ Vary the length of each piece of string from 6-12 inches. ☺ Thread a piece of string through or around each item. ☺ Make a tight knot around the object. ☺ Attach the other end of the string to the bottom of the coat hanger. ☺ Tie the rest of your items in the same way to the coat hanger. The more the merrier! ☺ Once you are done, hang your wind chimes near an open window or outside, and enjoy the jingle.

Common Scents

Chamomile: Calms

Cinnamon: Calms a queasy stomach

Lavender: Calms

Lemon/orange: Invigorates, helps you concentrate

Peppermint: Increases alertness

Pine: Stimulates

Rose: Calms, evens out your mood

Rosemary: Stimulates

Vanilla: Comforts

Rockin' Room Freshener

Basil gives you energy, lifts your spirits, and helps you focus. It's a good thing to sniff when you're doing your homework! Orange also smells delicious and can really perk you up.

Find an old spray bottle with a pump. A plastic hairspray bottle will work well. (But be sure to clean it out with hot water and soap and then rinse with cold water before filling with your new freshener.) ◎ Pour the distilled water into your bottle. ◎ Add the drops of basil and orange. ◎ Screw on the top and shake well. ◎ Spritz the air and enjoy the refreshing scent! ◎ When the room freshener is used up, clean the bottle. Also try making new blends with different scents.

SPA SUPPLIES

1/2 cup distilled water
3 drops basil essential oil
3 drops orange essential
   oil (you can also
   use mandarin or
   lemon oils)

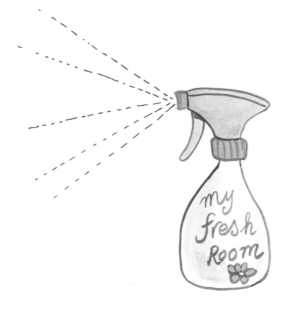

SPA PRINCESS

The time has come to treat your friends like royalty! Give each other fun names like Princess, Duchess, Queen, Baroness, Czarina, Empress, and Countess. Make crowns out of paper. Tell them that their every wish is your command. Instruct each friend to sit upon a throne (a.k.a. a chair) and put her feet up. Give her a Regal Reflexology Massage and an Imperial Pedicure.

And the best part is ... when the *spa*rty's over, your friends will bow down to you in thanks!

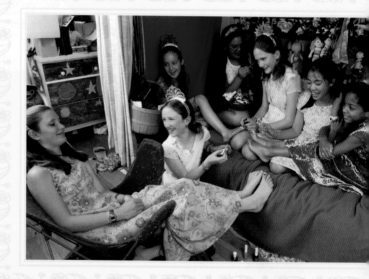

ROYAL ROLL-UPS

This stately snack is a snap to make. You mustn't keep the royalty waiting!

What you'll need (for the blintzes):
1 1/4 cups all-purpose flour
1/4 teaspoon salt
1 cup milk
3 eggs
4 tablespoons butter, melted
Powdered sugar

What you'll need (for the filling):
1 small tub of whipped
   cream cheese
1 jar of jam (try raspberry or
   boysenberry)

Combine all the blintz ingredients in a blender and blend until smooth. Pour the batter into a bowl. Put a large, nonstick pan on the stove over medium heat. Spray the pan with nonstick cooking spray. When the pan is hot, pour 1/4 cup of the batter into the pan. Swirl the batter to form a thin layer by tilting the skillet in a circular motion. Cook for two to four minutes, or until the edges start to curl slightly. Using a spatula, flip the blintz. (Careful, it's hot!) Cook for another one to two minutes. Remove the blintz from the pan using a spatula. Lay blintzes on top of each other on a plate. Place the plate of blintzes on the counter next to the whipped cream cheese and the jam. Put one blintz on the work surface. Spread a thin layer of whipped cream cheese all over the entire surface of the blintz. Place another blintz on top of the layer of whipped cream cheese and spread the new blintz with a thin layer of jam. Grab the bottom blintz and roll everything into a spiral and cut in half. Place each half on a plate and sprinkle with powdered sugar.

Makes eight blintzes.

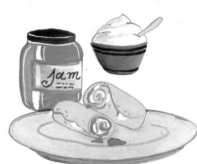

Spa
Specialities

SPA EATS

ROYAL ROLL-UPS

SPA TREATS

REGAL REFLEXOLOGY
MASSAGE

IMPERIAL PEDICURE

Stress Points:

Big toe: Brain and headaches

Tips of toes: Sinus

Arch: Stomach and digestion

Heel: Pelvis and rear

Area below second and third toe: Eye

Area below fourth and pinky toe: Ear

Inside edge of foot: Spine

Outside top edge of foot: Shoulder

Outside lower edge of foot: Hip

Regal Reflexology Massage

Reflexology is more than just a fancy way of saying foot rub. Students of this science believe that points on the foot are linked to different parts of your body. So with a little kneading and pressing, you can feel better all over. A good reflexology massage involves pressing your thumb into different stress points on the foot for several seconds at a time. So find a clean-footed friend and take turns massaging each other's tootsies. Be sure to take deep breaths during the massage and try not to be ticklish!

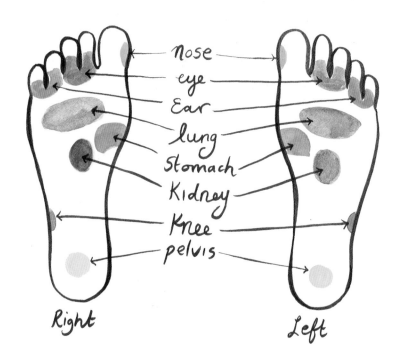

nose
eye
Ear
lung
Stomach
Kidney
Knee
pelvis

Right   Left

Imperial Pedicure

Give your feet the royal treatment! Start by washing your feet with soapy water, and then let 'em soak for a few minutes. Rub heels gently with a pumice stone and pat feet dry with a hand towel. Shape each nail with an emery board. File the tops straight across, rounding each slightly at the edges. Massage scented lotion into each foot. Dip a cotton ball into nail polish remover and wipe any excess lotion from each toenail. Paint your toes with colored nail polish. Wait 5–10 minutes and carefully place the stickers on the big toenails. If you are feeling crazy, sticker every nail! Preserve your handiwork by painting toenails with a topcoat of clear nail polish. Let dry for 10-15 minutes and then stick feet in a bowl of cold water to help the polish set and harden.

SPA SUPPLIES

Soapy water in large bowl
Hand towel
Pumice stone
Emery board
Scented lotion
Nail polish remover
Cotton balls
1 bottle of clear nail polish
1 bottle of brightly-
  colored nail polish
Sheet of small sparkly
  stickers

Hurrah SPA!

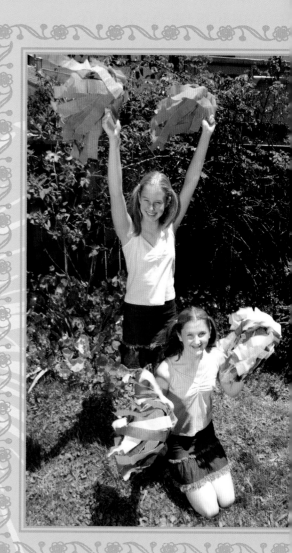

Forget about those nightmare gym classes at school. Sweating it spa style is a whole different type of workout. Now, getting fit can be fun – and fabulous! Get your lungs pumping by throwing an energy-boosting *sparty* for you and your closest friends. Jump, scream, kick, and get your heart racing as you perform favorite old-school cheers (or make up your own!). When you're all warmed up, treat yourself to some tasty chili and then cool down with a lemony body splash.

JUMPING CHILI BEAN SOUP

Put a little pep in your step with this protein-packed soup.

1/4 cup vegetable oil
1 onion, chopped
3 teaspoons chili powder
1 teaspoon cumin
1/2 6-ounce can tomato paste
1 14-ounce can diced tomatoes
2 cups water
2 15-ounce cans kidney
   beans, drained
1 teaspoon salt
1 cup grated cheddar cheese
2 green onions, chopped

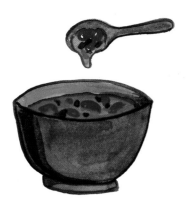

Heat oil in a large soup pan over medium heat. Add the chopped onions and cook until soft and slightly golden, stirring frequently. Add chili powder, cumin, tomato paste, tomatoes, water, beans, and salt. Simmer without a lid, stirring every few minutes, until the chili is thick (about 20 minutes). Carefully ladle the chili into bowls. Serve with grated cheddar cheese and green onions on top for garnish.

Makes four servings.

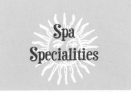

Spa Specialities

SPA EATS

JUMPING CHILI BEAN SOUP

SPA TREATS

HEARTY CHEER

CITRUS BODY SPLASH

Hearty Cheer

Cheering is an awesome way to give your lungs and body a workout. And it's way more physical than you might think. Done correctly, cheerleading takes hard work, training, and skill. But whether you're a seasoned squad member or just out for some fun, all that jumping around is sure to get your blood pumping.

Cut a bunch of colorful construction (or crepe) paper sheets into inch wide-strips. ◎ Bunch them together, then tape one end together. ◎ Finish off with a pretty ribbon, and you've got a set of personalized pom-poms. ◎ Now, get your squad together and create a cheer routine— complete with words, music, and moves! Feel free to cheer for whatever you like: your school, your town, your friendships— anything goes! ◎ Incorporate jumping jacks, kicks, funky dance moves, hip bumps, jumps, and lots of precision arm movements into your cheers. And don't forget to wear ultra-cute (but comfy) clothing, good athletic shoes, and stretch thoroughly before starting.

SPA SUPPLIES

Colored construction
 (or crepe) paper
Safety scissors
Scotchtape®
Ribbon

Citrus Body Splash

Lemons aren't just for lemonade. They can clean and soften skin. They also smell great and can energize a tired body. Create an all-over body splash that will have you jumping for joy!

SPA SUPPLIES

1 cup distilled water
Juice of 1 lemon
Spray bottle
Unscented face
  moisturizer

Find an old spray bottle with a pump. (Plastic hair spray bottles work great.) Scrub clean with hot soapy water and rinse. ☺ Squeeze out the juice of one whole lemon. ☺ Pour the juice and distilled water into your spray bottle, shake well, and spritz all over for a pick-me-up. ☺ Follow with a light coat of unscented face moisturizer. ☺ Shake well before each use and store in a cool, dark place (like the fridge). ☺ Toss out any leftover spray after two weeks. You don't want to smell like a sourpuss!

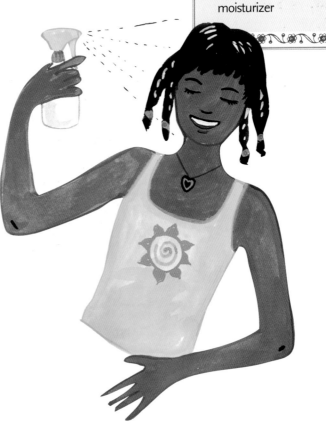

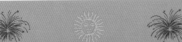

HEART SPA

Don't wait for a special occasion to show your love! And we're not talking about showing your affection for that unrequited crush that drives you bonkers. We're talking about your best girlfriends. You know, the ones you giggle, gossip, and gab with day in and day out. Invite them over for an extra-special *spa*rty to show them just how much you appreciate their friendship. Think pink (and red) and make everything pretty by having lots of fresh-cut flowers and heart-shaped treats. Play DJ and spin a mix of girl-power themed songs to set a rockin' and rosy mood.

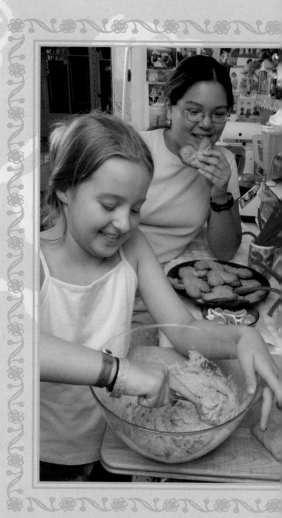

SWEET HEART COOKIES

Eat your heart out! These oatmeal cookies are the perfect hearty snacks for your guests.

1/2 cup butter, softened
1/4 cup sugar
1/4 cup brown sugar
1 tablespoon molasses
1 egg
1 cup flour

1 cup oatmeal
1/2 cup pecans, chopped
1 teaspoon baking powder
1/2 teaspoon baking soda
1/2 teaspoon cinnamon
1/4 teaspoon salt

Preheat the oven to 350 degrees. ❧ Cream together the butter, sugar, brown sugar, and molasses with a wooden spoon (or a hand mixer) in a large bowl. ❧ Add the egg and continue to blend together. ❧ In another bowl, combine the flour, oatmeal, pecans, baking powder, baking soda, cinnamon, and salt. ❧ Add the flour mixture to the butter mixture and stir to combine. ❧ Put the dough in the refrigerator for 10 minutes. ❧ Take the dough out of the refrigerator and set on the counter with a cookie sheet. ❧ Take one teaspoon of the dough and roll it between your hands to make a tiny log of dough about two to three inches long. Make another log and use both sections to create each side of the heart shape. Pinch sides together to connect and place on cookie sheet. ❧ Repeat until the cookie sheet is full, leaving about four inches between each cookie. ❧ Bake for 8-10 minutes. ❧ Carefully remove the cookie sheet from the oven and let cool on a wire rack. Using a spatula, carefully transfer the cookies to a serving plate.

Makes 25-30 treats.

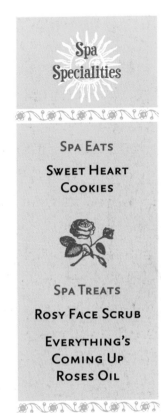

Spa Specialities

SPA EATS

SWEET HEART COOKIES

SPA TREATS

ROSY FACE SCRUB

EVERYTHING'S COMING UP ROSES OIL

Rosy Face Scrub

SPA SUPPLIES

2 tablespoons oatmeal
1 tablespoon warm water
1 washcloth

Oatmeal does double duty. It draws out dirt and oil from your skin and it gets rid of dry skin. Add warm water to the oatmeal until you make a thick paste. ◎ Smear paste onto a clean face. ◎ Rub it gently over your cheeks, forehead, and chin. Avoid getting any of the goop in your eyes. ◎ Leave the mask on for 5-7 minutes, rinse with warm water, and pat dry. ◎ Take a look in the mirror and check out your rosy cheeks!

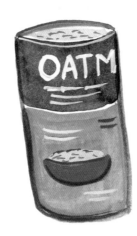

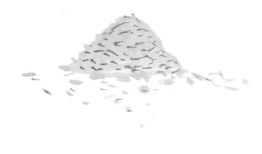

Everything's Coming Up Roses Oil

SPA SUPPLIES

2 tablespoons
  sweet almond oil
2 drops of rose
  essential oil
Small glass bottle

Pour sweet almond oil into a small glass bottle and then add the drops of rose oil. Put the cap (or dropper) on the bottle and shake well. Rub a few drops on your pulse points – temples, neck, wrists, inside of elbows, backs of knees, ankles. Breathe deeply and enjoy smelling like a rose!

For extra fun: Use your rosy potion to cast a love spell. Grab a crystal or sparkly object, such as a necklace or earring. Head outside and, under the light of the moon, hold up your crystal and chant a magical spa poem:

> Spa light, spa bright,
>
> First star I see tonight
>
> Wish I may, wish I might
>
> Catch (insert your crush's name)'s eye in daylight.

Wear the crystal and the potion the next time you plan on seeing him. He won't be able to take his eyes (or his nose) off you!

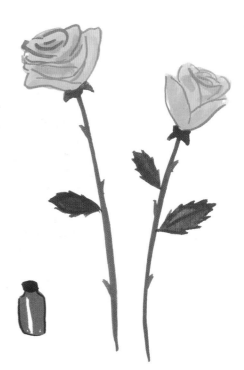

BEACH-BLANKET SPA

Bring the beach home with this sun, shell, and sand spa. If the weather's nice, hold your *spa*rty outside. Ask your guests to sport beach gear and bring along sunglasses, towels, and sunscreen. For a stylish look, drape a scarf (or sarong) around your body and tuck a flower behind your ear. Lounge around on retro beach blankets and eat tropical fruit. Create cool seashell candles to decorate your room or backyard. Enjoy a sandy foot scrub and get ready to hula the day away!

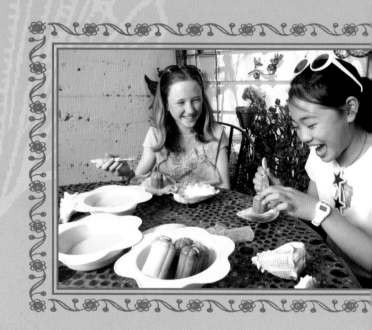

TROPICAL FREEZE

This exotic treat will cool you down as your *spa*rty heats up.

4 cups tropical or juicy fruit, cubed

1 teaspoon lemon or limejuice

1 tablespoon sugar

Try mangoes, peaches, strawberries, papayas, pineapples, melons,
or kiwis. (Or any creative combo you like!)

Peel, seed, trim, or pit the fruit of your choice and chop it into cubes.
Put the four cups of fruit cubes into a bag (that can be sealed) or
a container and put it in the freezer until frozen. Carefully put the
frozen fruit, lemon juice, and sugar into the food processor.
Close the lid and blend until smooth. If the fruit seems
too frozen to blend, let the fruit defrost
for 15 minutes, then try again.
Carefully scoop the
tropical freeze out of the
food processor and serve.

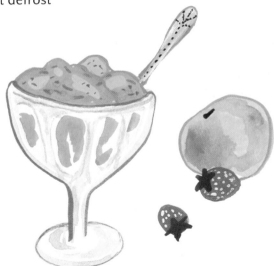

Makes four servings.

Spa
Specialities

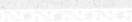

SPA EATS
TROPICAL FREEZE

SPA TREATS
SEASHELL CANDLES
SANDY FOOT SCRUB

SPA SUPPLIES

A clam shell (or similarly shaped shell big enough to hold a tea candle)

Tea (or short) candle

Glitter glue

Sand (or salt)

Seashell Candles

Ah, the beach! It's more than just a place to swim, sunbath, hang with friends or family, and create great summertime memories. There's something magical about it. For many, it's a sacred spot to getaway, relax, and think. That may be why seashells (also called "jewels of the sea") are so popular. Some people have been collecting them since childhood. Others use them as home decorations or give them to loved ones as gifts. And still others use them to get crafty, making them into jewelry, wreaths, lamps, and more! Now you too can bring a little bit of the beach home with this shell candle!

Fill the bottom of a shell with a layer of sand. ◎ Roll the sides of your candle in glitter glue so that it's sparkly on the outside. ◎ Let dry. ◎ Place your candle in the shell. ◎ The sand will help anchor the candle in the shell so it doesn't move around. ◎ Place in a safe spot and ask your parents if you can light your new seashell candle!

Sandy Foot Scrub

Ever notice how good your feet feel after a day of walking along the beach? Sand softens rough spots and exercises the muscles in your feet and legs. Now you can enjoy the benefits of sand with an energizing foot scrub.

Mix all the ingredients together in a small bowl. ◎ Take half of the mixture and rub it onto your right foot. Pay particular attention to the sole of each foot and don't forget the area between each toe! Repeat on left foot. ◎ Rinse thoroughly in a bowl of warm water (or under a faucet) and slip on an old pair of socks to seal in the moisture. Your feet will feel beachy clean in no time!

SPA SUPPLIES

2 tablespoons sand

2 tablespoons canola or olive oil

6 drops rosemary or peppermint oil

SPA HAS SPRUNG

After a long, dreary winter, shake off the cold weather with some of the best things spring has to offer. Eat fresh fruit, drink lots of water, and treat yourself to a healthy flower salad. Clear your head with an herbal eye pillow or clean your skin with a delicious papaya mask. Birds will sing, bees will buzz, and flowers will bloom. Swear!

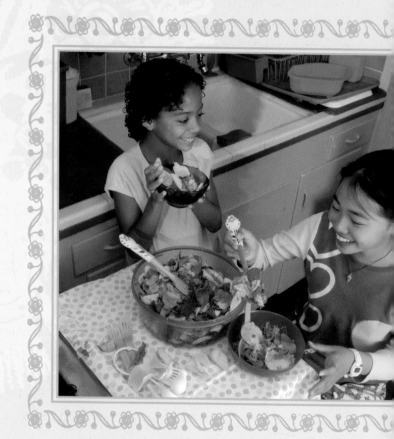

FLOWER POWER SALAD

Some flowers taste as nice as they smell, so dig into this colorful salad mix.

What you'll need (for the salad):
4 cups of tightly-packed, chopped lettuce
1 carrot, peeled and grated
1/2 cucumber, peeled and sliced
1 cup cherry tomatoes, cut in half
1/4 cup mixed herbs like basil, mint, parsley, chives, or chervil
1/4 cup mixed petals from edible flowers like nasturtium, marigolds, chamomile, dandelions, lilac, queen anne's lace, roses, and violets (You can usually find these in the produce section or get them from a garden where NO pesticides are used and wash them well.)

What you'll need (for the dressing):
6 tablespoons olive oil
2 tablespoons red wine vinegar
1 teaspoon Dijon mustard
1/2 teaspoon sugar
1/4 teaspoon salt
1/4 teaspoon pepper

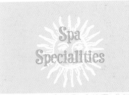

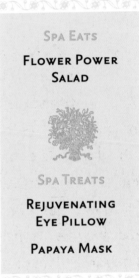

Spa Specialties

SPA EATS
FLOWER POWER SALAD

SPA TREATS
REJUVENATING EYE PILLOW
PAPAYA MASK

In a large bowl add the lettuce, carrot, cucumber, cherry tomatoes, herbs, and flowers. In a small jar with a tight-fitting lid, combine the oil, vinegar, Dijon mustard, sugar, salt, and pepper. Shake well until blended. Pour half the salad dressing over the lettuce mix and toss. Taste a piece of lettuce to see if you would like more dressing. Add more if you want and toss again.

Makes four servings.

Rejuvenating Eye Pillow

Eye pillows are a great way to rest tired eyes. All you need is an old T-shirt and a little creativity. Try to use colored tees, if you can. (Be sure to get an okay from your parents before you cut up any shirts.) One shirt will make two to four eye pillows.

Cut the sleeve (as close to the shoulder seam as possible) off the shirt. You should now have a "tube" of tee material. Knot one end of the tube. ◎ Mix the rice and lavender in a small bowl. ◎ Fill your T-shirt tube with the mixture. Tightly knot the other end. (The pillow should be about six inches long between knots.) ◎ Trim off any straggles or extra material. It should feel soft and floppy rather than stuffed tight. The rice should move around inside the pillow. ◎ Tie ribbons around the knots. Your herbal eye pillow is ready for action! ◎ Lie down, close your lids, and place the pillow over your eyes. Breathe deeply. Rest under the gentle pressure of the pillow.

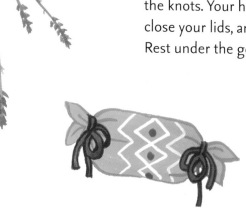

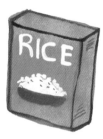

Papaya Mask

Fresh papaya is a great way to get rid of winter's dry flaky skin. And it smells really yummy! ◎ Peel the papaya and remove seeds. ◎ Mash the fruit of the papaya with a fork into a bowl. ◎ Spread a small handful of the fruit mush on your face. ◎ Kick back and rest for 10 minutes while the papaya goes to work. ◎ Wash off with warm water and blot your face dry with a washcloth. Now sit back, lick your fingers, and feel fabulous.

SPA SUPPLIES

1/4 ripe papaya
Small bowl
Washcloth

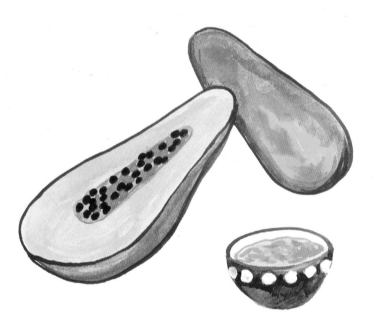

BATHING BEAUTY SPA

It's skin to the wind during this bath party. Bathing has been serious business for thousands of years. In ancient Rome and Greece, men and women went to public baths. While they visited with friends, they cleansed their bodies in the large pools of steamy and chilled water. Even with all of today's high-tech treatments and spendy products, it's still a great way to unwind, pamper, and heal both your body and mind.

Set up your spa in the bathroom. (Make sure your family doesn't need to use it during your party!) Get a portable stereo and stock up on fresh bath towels, fashion mags, and tasty snacks in plastic glasses (placed within easy reach, of course!). Slip into cute bathing suits and fuzzy robes, and finally – best of all – take turns soaking in the tub, drawing a new bath for each spa guest.

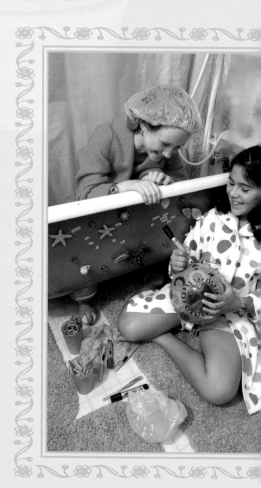

SPABERRY SHAKE

Keep cool and hydrated with this vitamin-packed shake. Don't forget the straw!

12 strawberries
1 tablespoon sugar
5 ice cubes
1/2 cup low-fat milk
Two straws

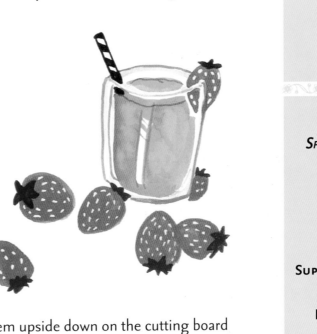

Cut the green tops off 10 of the strawberries, then cut them in half. Put the cut strawberries, sugar, ice cubes, and milk in the blender. Blend until smooth. Pour the blend into glasses. Cut the remaining two strawberries almost in half by turning them upside down on the cutting board and slicing them from the red tip ALMOST all the way to the green leaf – but not through it. Perch the strawberry on the side of the glass by slipping the two halves of the strawberry onto the rim. Get two straws, serve, and enjoy!

Makes two eight-ounce shakes.

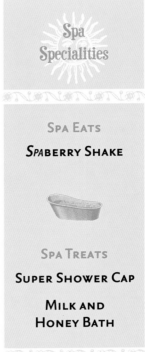

Spa
Specialities

SPA EATS
SPABERRY SHAKE

SPA TREATS
SUPER SHOWER CAP

MILK AND HONEY BATH

SPA SUPPLIES

Solid-colored shower caps
Permanent markers
Soccer or basketball

Super Shower Cap

For *sparty*-goers who want to take a soak without drenching their do, a Super Shower Cap is just the answer. Get cheap, solid-colored shower caps at the drugstore. Put each cap on a basketball (or something similar in size) to make it easier to decorate. Then create designs on the caps with permanent markers. Flowers, raindrops, and polka dots are all fun ideas.

Milk and Honey Bath

Live like a queen! The beautiful Egyptian ruler Cleopatra soaked regularly in soothing milk baths. Honey draws moisture to the skin, so it's a great way to soften your body.

Mix the milk and honey together in a bowl. ◎ Fill the tub with warm water. ◎ Swirl in the milk and honey mixture. ◎ Tuck your hair under your Super Shower Cap and set your *Spa*berry Shake within reach. (Don't forget the straw!) ◎ Step into the tub, lean back, and sink into your yummy bath.

SPA SUPPLIES

1 quart whole milk
1/4 cup honey

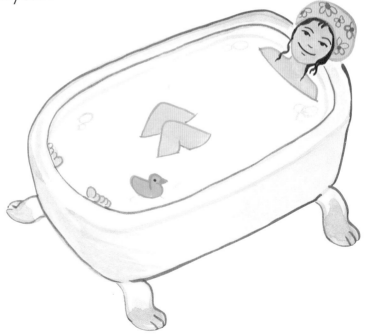

SPA BUCKS

Remember setting up lemonade stands and making cupcakes for the bake sale? Now that you know how to make so many mind, body, and soul treats, it's time to expand those childhood dreams of becoming a big business tycoon. Use what you've learned in this book (and all your other great ideas), and go public! Save major bucks and give your creations as holiday gifts for friends and family. Or (even better), set up your very own bedroom boutique (or sidewalk shop), sell your luxury goods, and pocket the profit.

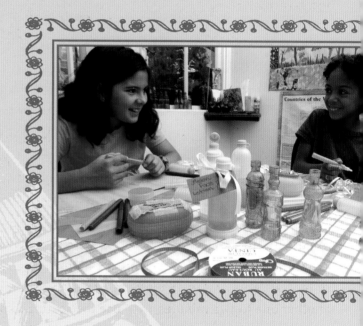

SILVER-DOLLAR PANCAKES

Kick off your new business with these prosperous pancakes.

1 cup all-purpose flour
2 teaspoons baking powder
2 tablespoons sugar
1/2 teaspoon salt
1 cup milk
2 tablespoons butter, melted
1 egg
1 teaspoon vanilla
1 cup blueberries, chopped strawberries, or banana rounds

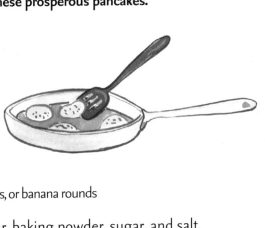

In a medium bowl, mix the flour, baking powder, sugar, and salt.
🌿 In a large bowl, mix the milk, melted butter, egg, and vanilla.
🌿 Add the flour mixture to the milk mixture and blend until there
are no lumps. 🌿 Put a large, nonstick skillet on the stove over
medium heat. When the pan is hot, pour one tablespoon of the
batter into the pan to make a pancake. Add more pancakes to the
pan if there is room. 🌿 Cook until tiny bubbles appear on the top
of the pancakes, and then flip them over with a spatula. Cook for
another one to two minutes, then use the spatula to place the
pancakes on a serving plate. 🌿 Serve topped with butter and
syrup. Sprinkle blueberries, strawberries, and/or bananas on top.

Makes 20 medium-sized pancakes.

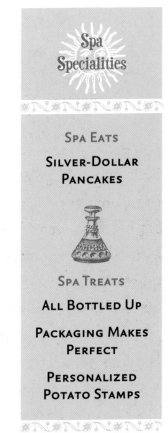

Mix and match words for inspiration!

Your name	Place
Awesome	Posh
Body	Potion
Calming	Relaxing
Designer	Shop
Face	Skin
Factory	Spa
Fruity	Stylish
Garden	Swank
Juicy	Sweet
Kitchen	Tasty
Lab	Treat
Luscious	Treatment
Mod	Ultimate
Oasis	Workshop
Palace	Yummy

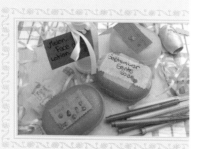

All Bottled Up

There are a lot of packaging options out there. Craft and health food stores have bottles and jars for storing your lotions and potions. You can also ask your mom to save food jars and containers as well as empty shampoo and lotion bottles. Clean them out and, with mom or dad's help, dip them in boiling water for a few seconds to sterilize them. They'll be as good as new.

Packaging Makes Perfect

You can create your own labels, tags, and stickers with glitter glue, gel (or metallic) pens, and whatever else you have on hand.

When it comes to naming your products, be as creative as you can. Include your name and words that incorporate your interests and hobbies. Also think about how the lotions smell and the way they make you feel.

Create a flyer that lists your products. Think about how much the ingredients cost when pricing your potions. Add in the cost of the bottle (or jar), and supplies you bought to create labels and tags. Write a description of each product and list all the yummy ingredients. Most products with fresh fruits and vegetables won't keep for more than a week or two so make these products fresh each time. Also, when using essential oils in products, store your bottles in a cool, dark place.

Personalized Potato Stamps

Raid the pantry for potatoes and make unique stamps for your products!

Peel and cut a potato into slices about 1/2 inch thick. ◎ Pat the slices of the potato with a paper towel.◎ Lay the potato slices on a cutting board. ◎ Press a cookie cutter into them as if you were cutting out dough for cookies. Try using star, heart, flower, sun, and moon cookie cutters. You now have potato stamps to use for your packaging! ◎ Press down firmly with your potato stamp on the inkpad. Try out your stamp on a scrap piece of paper. If you like the results, stamp away! ◎ Write out the name of the product, the date you made it, and any special instructions for use. Attach it to your jar or bottle.

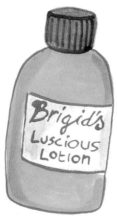

SPA SUPPLIES

1 potato per person
Potato peeler
Dinner knife
Cookie cutters in
    fun shapes
1 inkpad (color choice
    is yours!)
Sticky sheets of labels
    (or light-colored
    construction paper)
Hole puncher

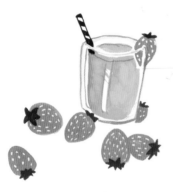
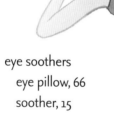

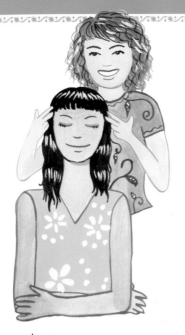

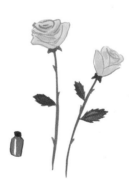

Thanks goes to everyone who participated in the creation, direction, and production of this book. We couldn't have done it without all of you!

Creative Directors
Hallie Warshaw
Tanya Napier

Writers
Erin Conley
Jennifer Worick

Recipe Writer
Katrina Hendriks

Graphic Designers
Tanya Napier
Hallie Warshaw

Photographer
Julie Brown

Illustrator
Annie Galvin

Editor
Erin Conley

Production Artist
Kristine Mudd

**Additional Production
and Photo Stylist**
Domini Dragoone

Special thanks to all the
SPA-TACULAR models:

Georgina Garcia

Louise Harrington

Rhianna Hixon

Sierra Hixon

Connie Johnson

Nina Krietzman

Amanda Minafo

Carrie Nattinger

Itai Brand-Thomas

Madeline Wayham

Mayton Xu

Photoshoot Home:

Special thanks to the Hixon family for letting us descend upon their lovely home for the photo shoot.

Created and produced by **Orange Avenue Publishing,** 599 Third Street, Suite 306, San Francisco, CA 94107

ABOUT THE CREATORS

Erin Conley is a freelance writer/editor who loves to be pampered. She lives in San Francisco, but makes it a habit to hit the spa wherever (and whenever) she can. Favorite spa treatments include: hot stone massages, green tea facials, and warm milk & lavender pedicures. She is proud to be a total *spa*rty animal.

Jennifer Worick is a writer, editor, and all-around spa fanatic and product junkie. She has written books on Nancy Drew, belly dancing, love, and action heroines. When she's stressed out by a deadline, she paints her toes, gives herself a facial, or splurges on a hot stone massage. Jennifer grew up on the shores of Lake Michigan and graduated from the University of Michigan. She now calls Philadelphia home.

Julie Brown enjoys photographing people - their lives and surroundings. One of her specialties is black-and-white documentary photography. Her photographs have been featured in various local and national publications, and this is her fourth children's book. Julie holds a Bachelor of Fine Arts from the Rochester Institute of Technology. She lives in Great Barrington, MA. Julie likes to relax in a hot sauna.

Annie Galvin can't decide if she's an illustrator who writes or a writer who illustrates. Making paper dolls and writing poems are a few of her favorite pastimes. Originally from Ireland, Annie lives in San Francisco with her husband, a painter who writes. Annie's favorite aromatherapy scents are lavender and lemon verbena.

Tanya Napier is a writer, designer and painter of teddy portraits. She has written for various publications in Boston and New York, and now works as a copywriter and graphic designer in San Francisco. Tanya grew up in England, not far from the lovely town of Bath. Not surprisingly, her favorite way to unwind is to take a tub (Epsom salt and rubber ducky included).

Hallie Warshaw loves children's books, bright colors, and dogs, especially her own, Baci. Before founding Orange Avenue Publishing in 1997, Hallie was a creative director and graphic designer in Hong Kong, Osaka, and New York. Hallie holds bachelor degrees from Clark University and the Rhode Island School of Design. She lives in San Francisco in a pastel yellow building that she wishes were bright orange. Hallie gets massages as often as possible.